I0721073

Dedicated to…

all the family,
friends and
medical workers
that supported
Isabella while
hospitalized late
Nov 2020 to late
Feb 2021 and to
ALL that have
supported her

thereafter!

**Now
for you, dearest
reader!**
This is not just a
book.

Oh no!

This is a learning
tool, written for
someone SMART like
you to share with
others!

As you read, be on the lookout for the following words,

- ☐ Lupus
- ☐ Flare
- ☐ Vitals
- ☐ Joint

Also take a look at who we get to meet...

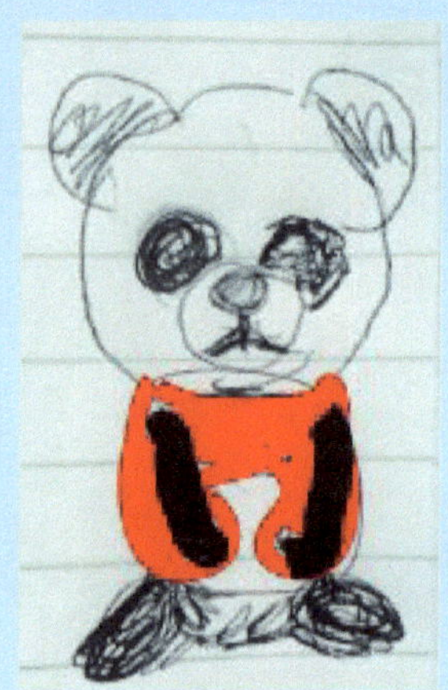

Daddy

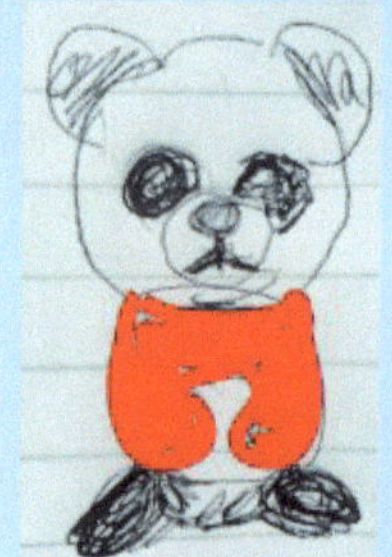

Tuto

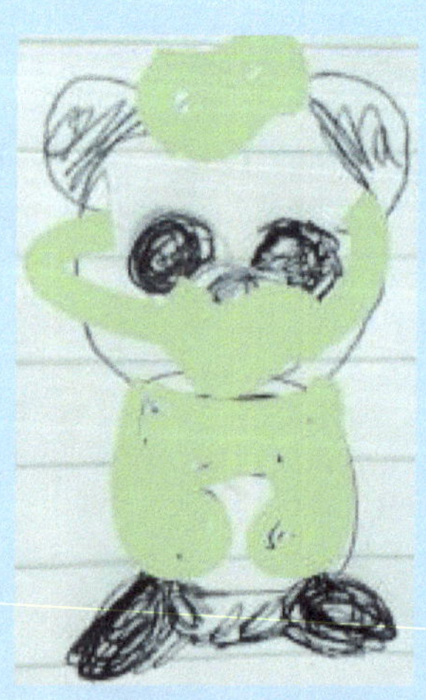

Nurse Rose

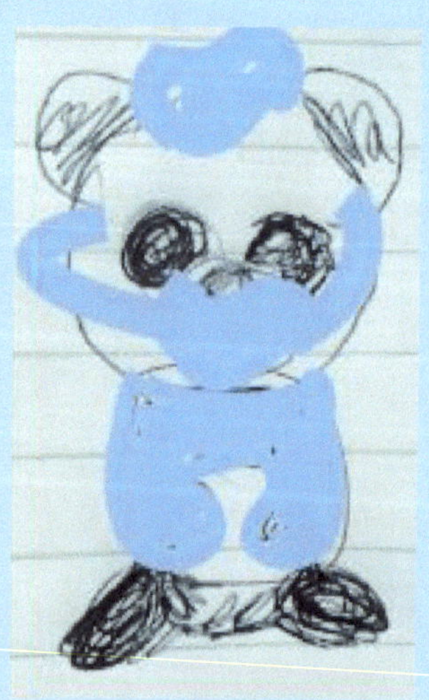

Dr.Simmons

Continue
now to
see where
*Tuto
Goes...*

Tuto Goes
for a Checkup

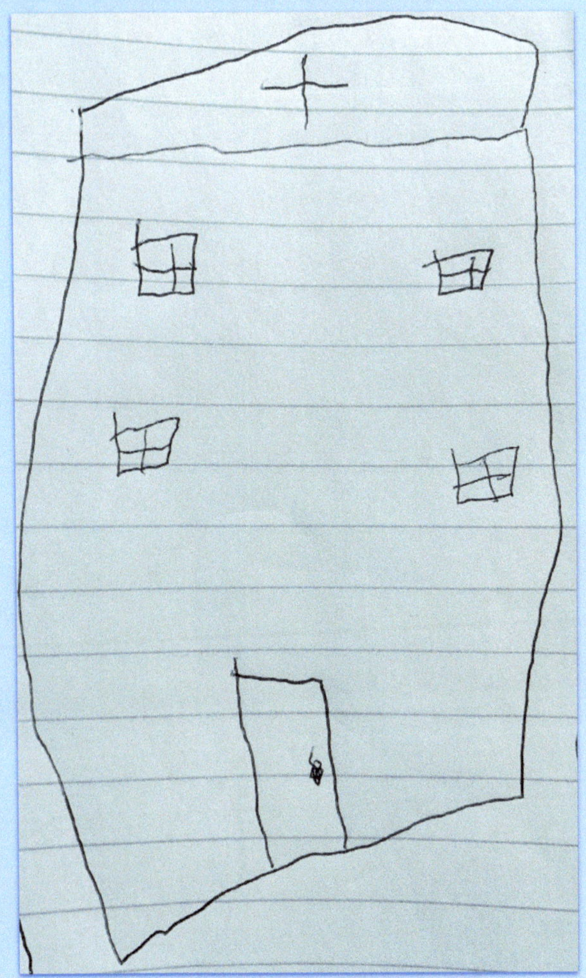

A Pediatric tale about Lupus

Written by Jasmine Casilla
Illustrated by Isabella Casilla

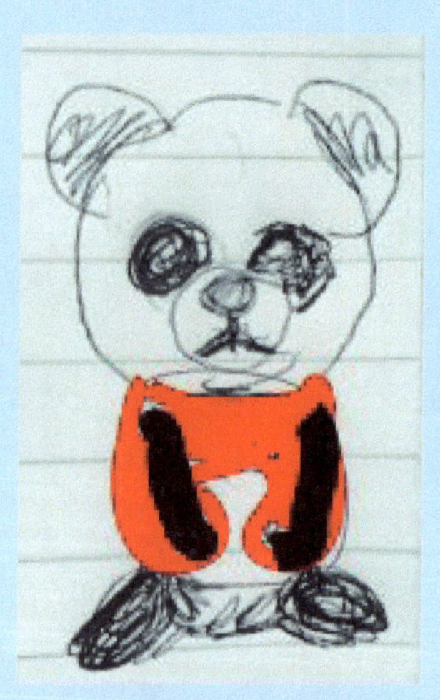

Good morning Tuto!

Are you ready for your **Lupus** checkup?

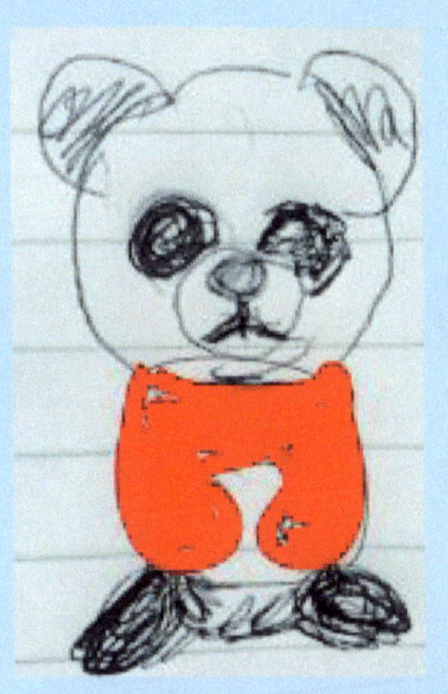

Yes, Daddy.

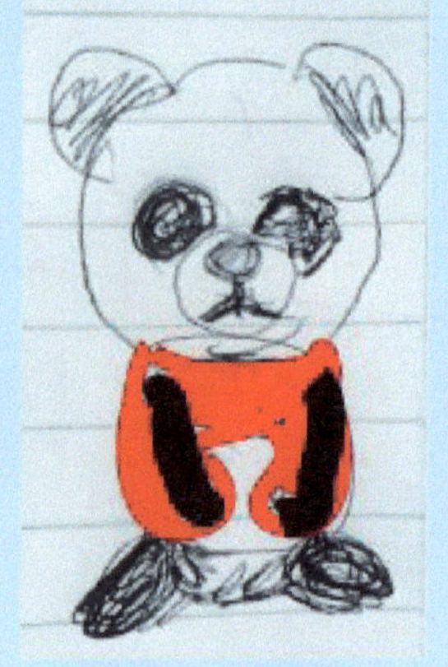

Ok, Tuto.

But before we
leave, we must put
on your sunscreen
for protection so
you don't have a
flare.

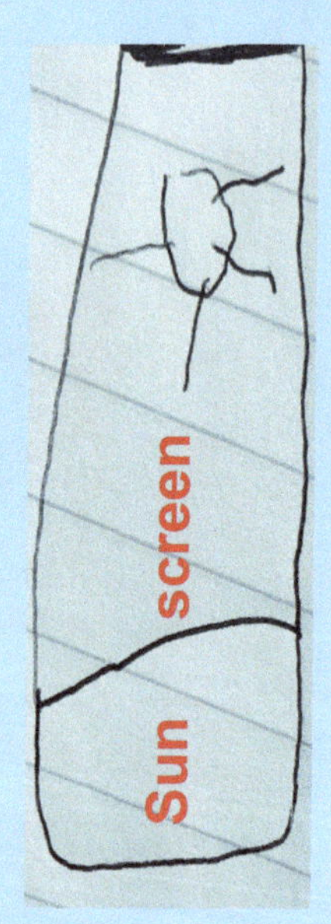

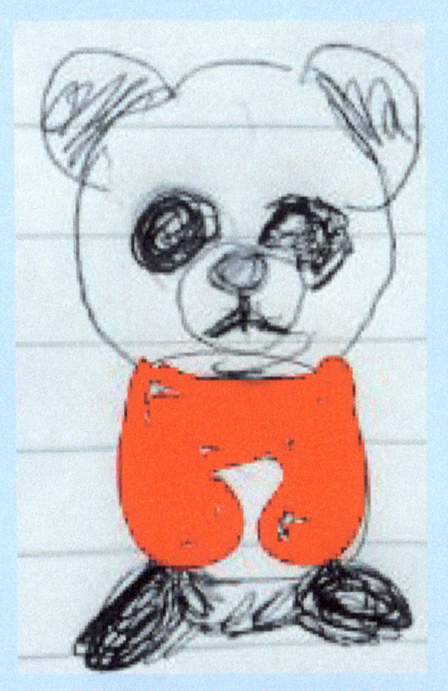

Daddy, what's a **flare**?

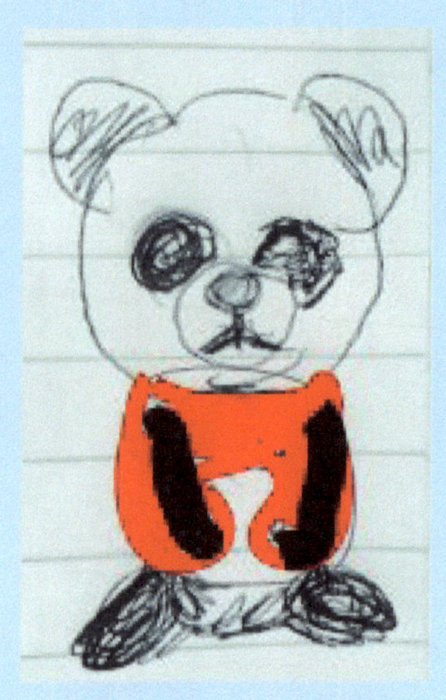

That's a GREAT question Tuto!

Sometimes with **Lupus**, you feel bad. You may have a fever, achy body or ouchies in your mouth.

We call those things a **flare**.

Does that make sense?

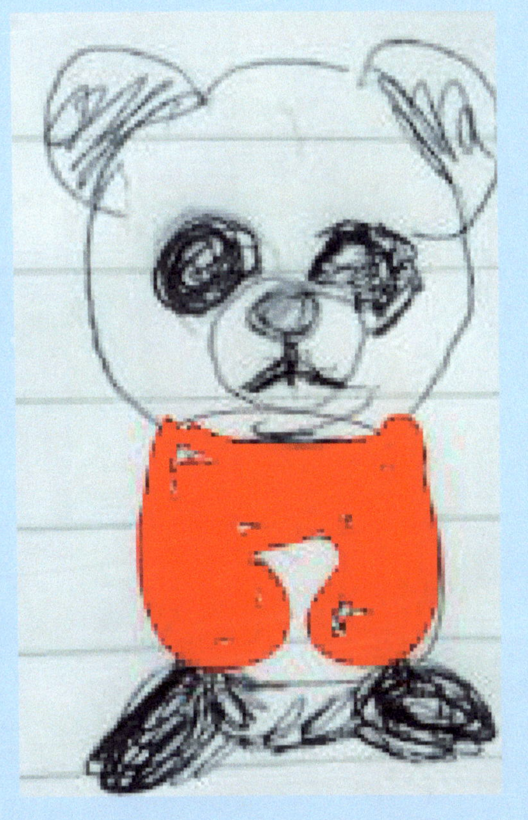

Yes, Daddy.

Doctor's office

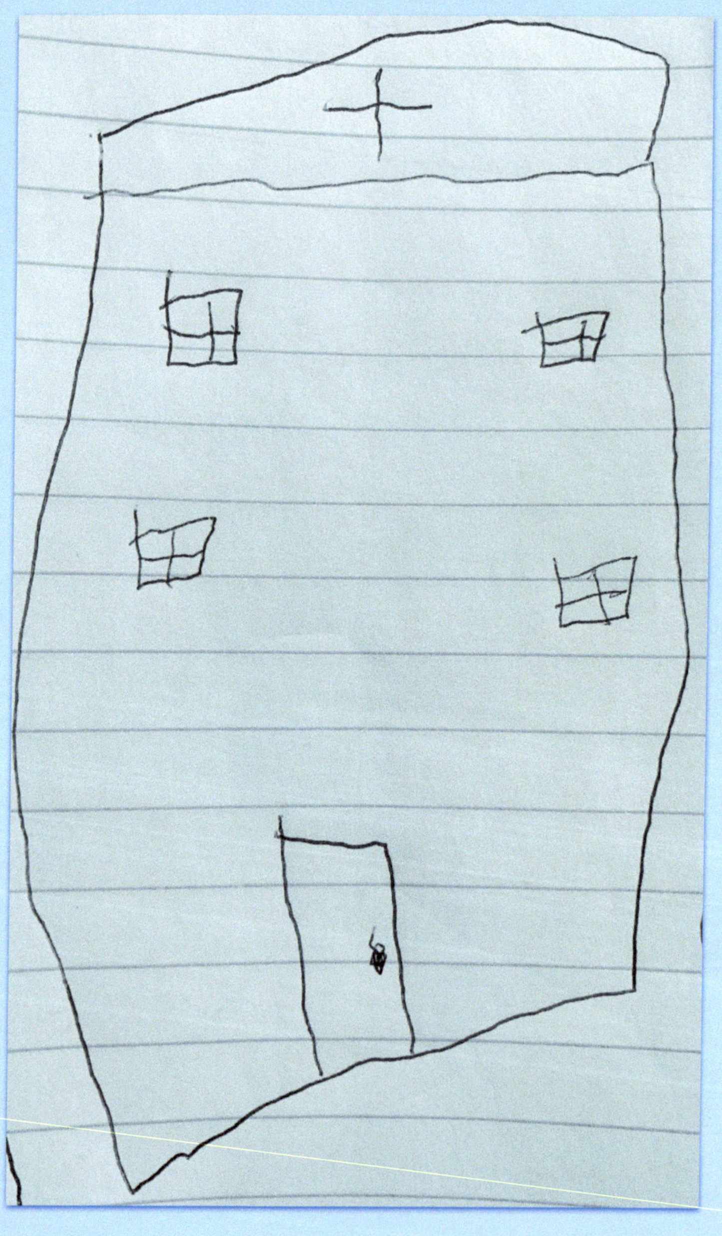

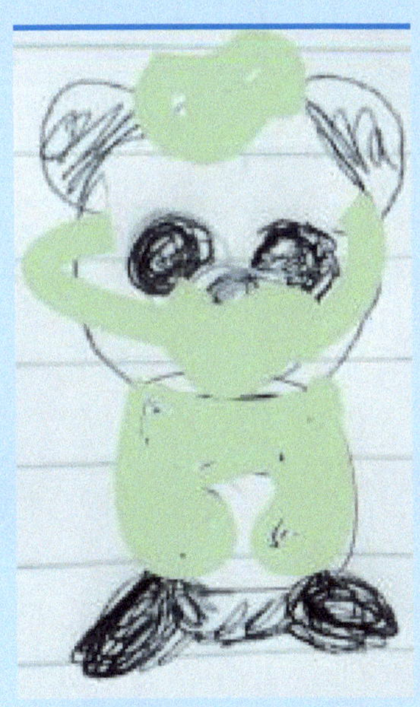

Hello, Tuto.

My name is Rose.

I will be your
nurse today.

.

May I check your
vitals, before the
doctor comes in?

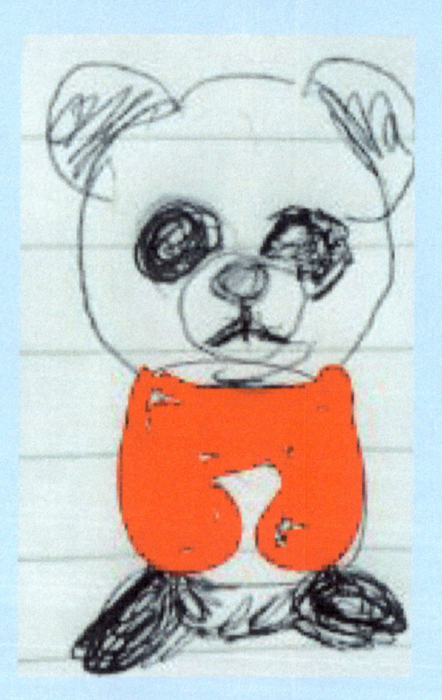

Tuto leans
over and
whispers,

"Daddy, What
are **vitals**?"

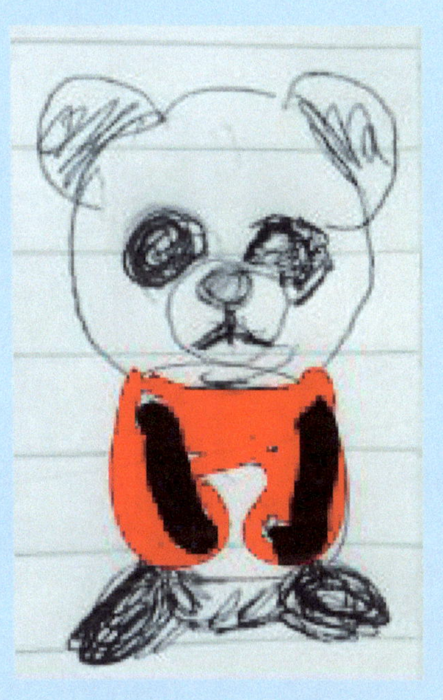

That's a great
question Tuto!

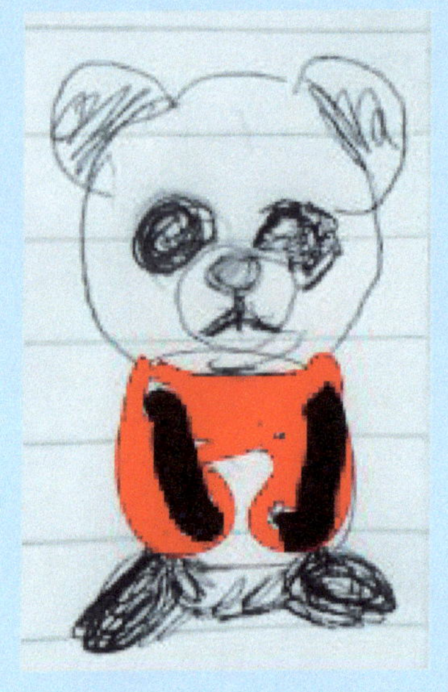

Vitals are all the important information that your doctor wants to know, like your temperature, blood pressure, weight and height.

Does that make sense?

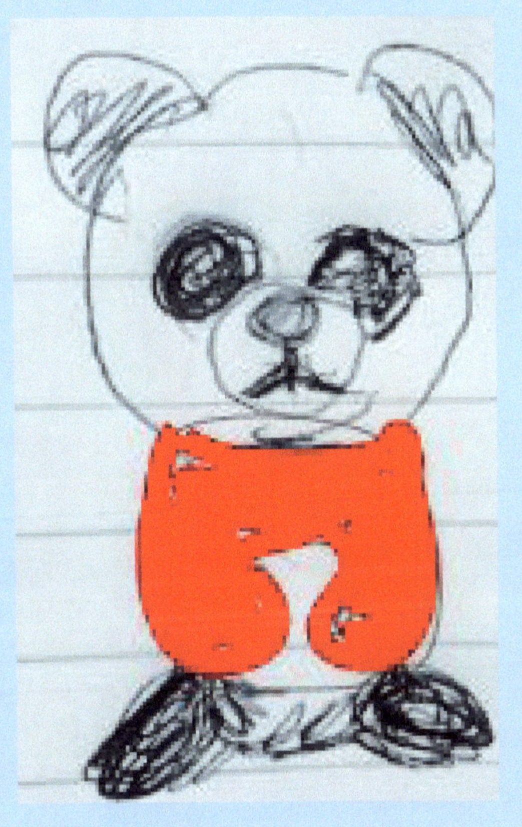

Yes, Daddy.

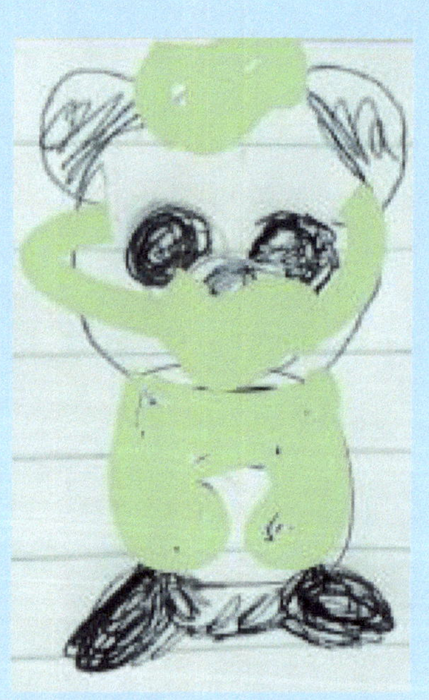

So, can I
check your
vitals
Tuto?

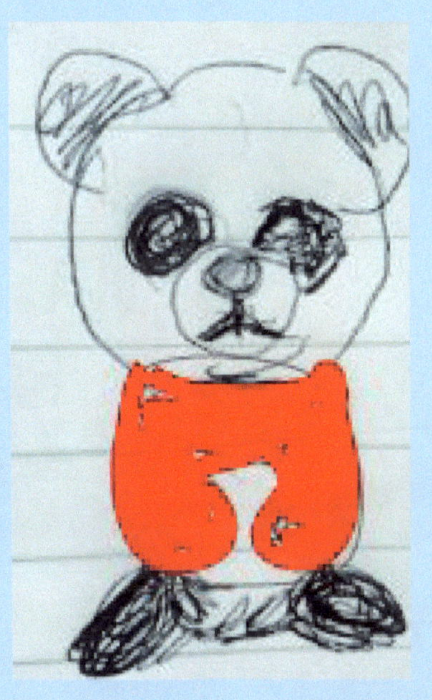

Yes,Nurse.

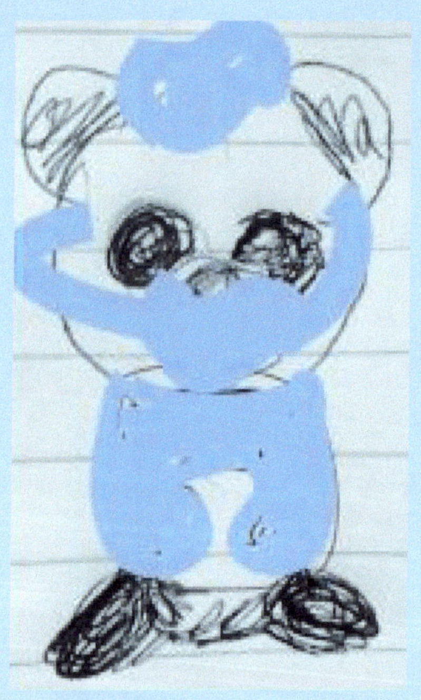

Hello Tuto,

I'm
Dr. Simmons.

Can I take a
listen to
your heart?

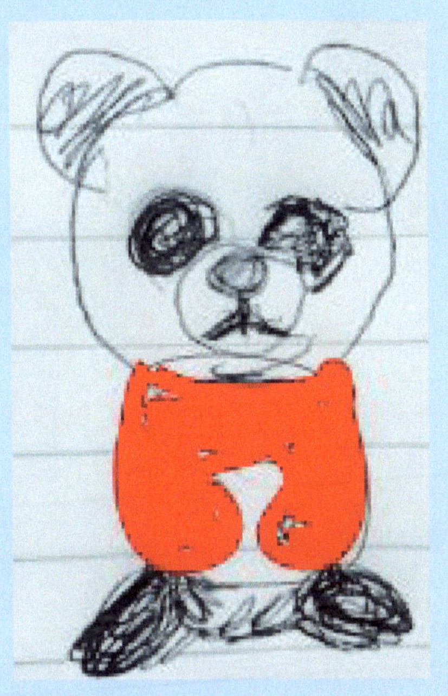

Yes, Doctor.

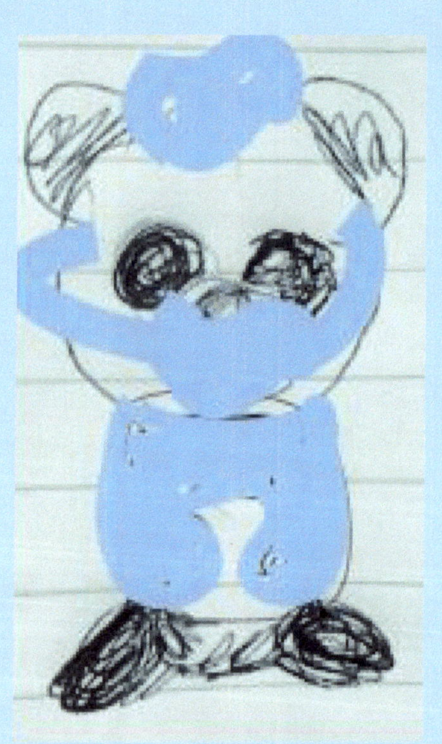

Can I take
a look in
your mouth,
to see if
you have
any
ouchies?

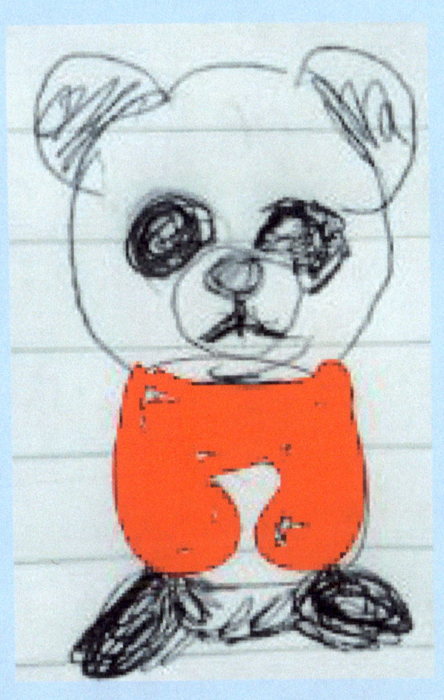

Yes,Doctor.

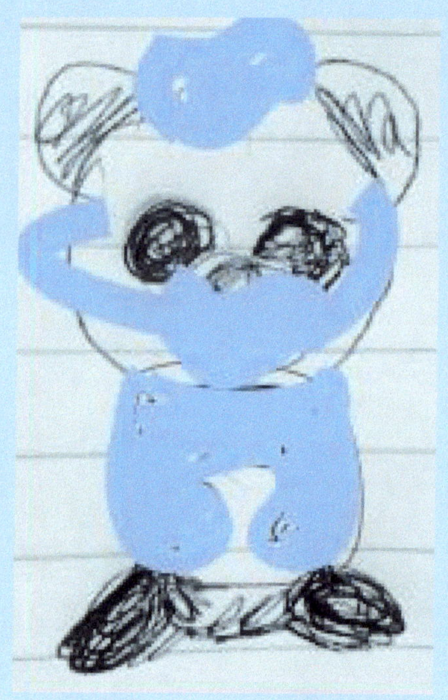

Everything is great so far!

Just one more thing Tuto.

Do you mind if I check your **joints** for ouchies?

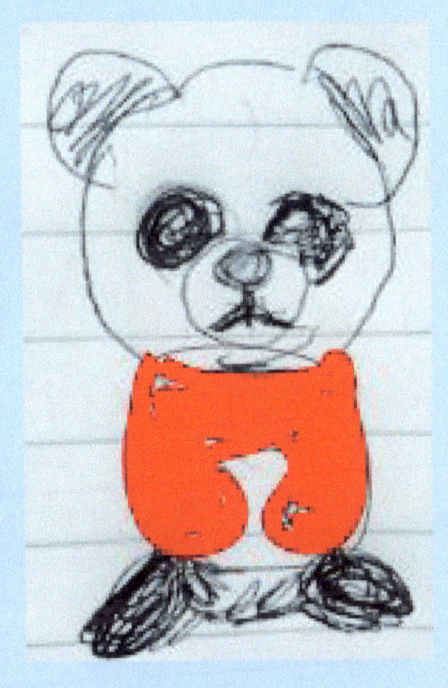

Tuto leans over and whispers,

"Daddy, what's a **joint**?"

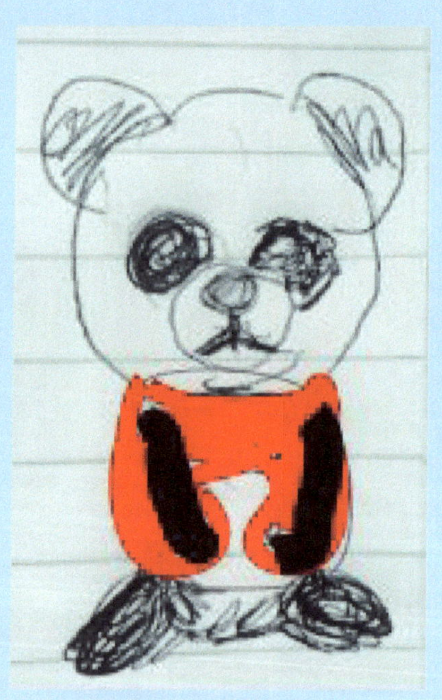

That's a
great
question
Tuto!

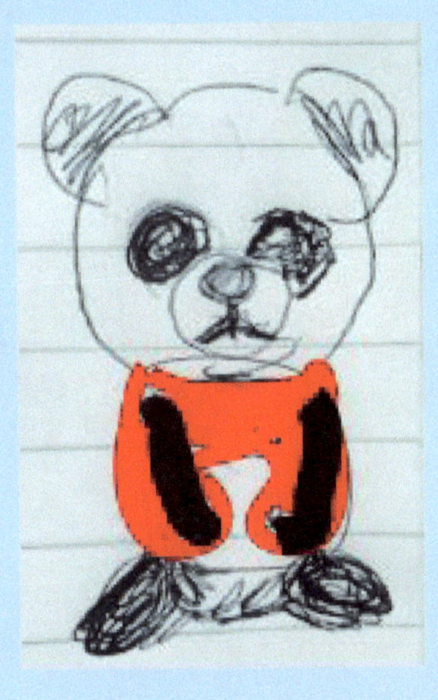

Joints are the spaces between the bones in your body.

They're in your knees and wrist and most bendy things, like your fingers and toes and your elbows.

Does that make sense?

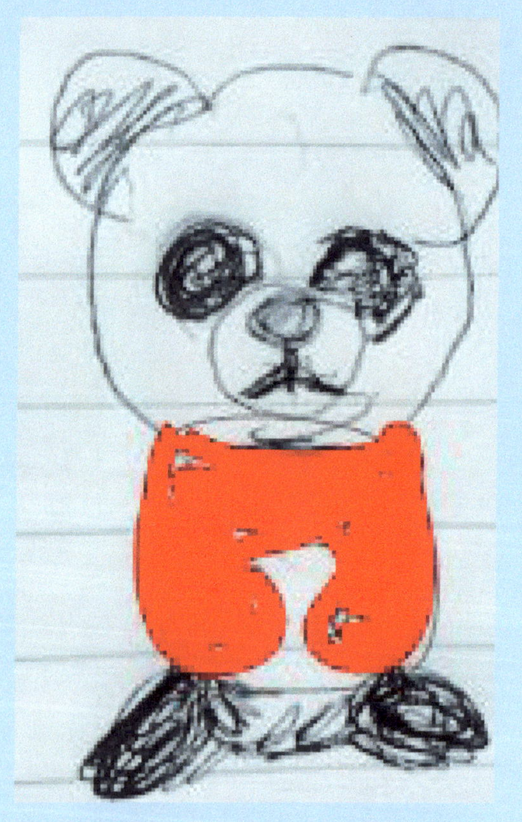

Yes, Daddy.

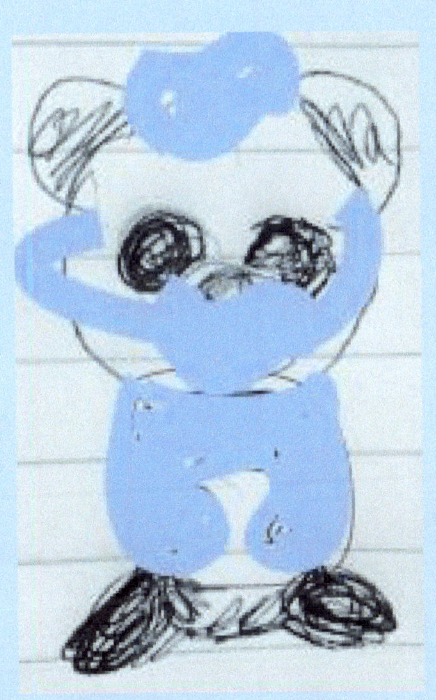

May I check
your **joints**
Tuto?

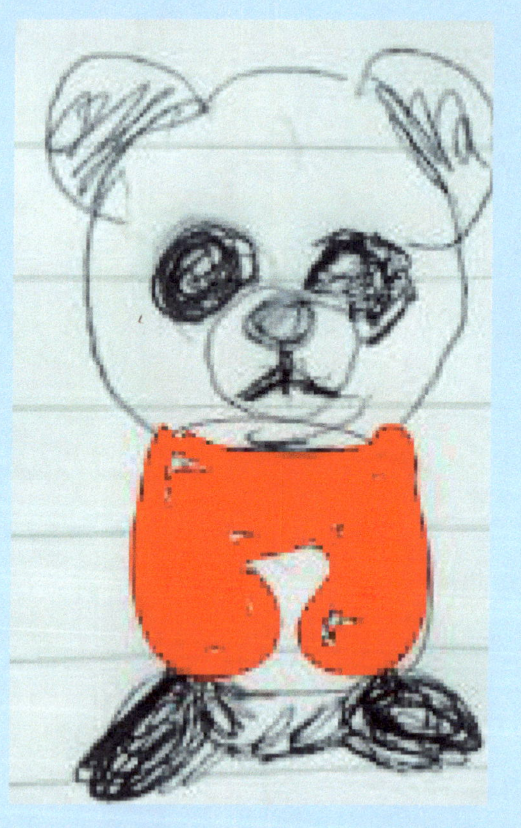

Yes, Doctor.

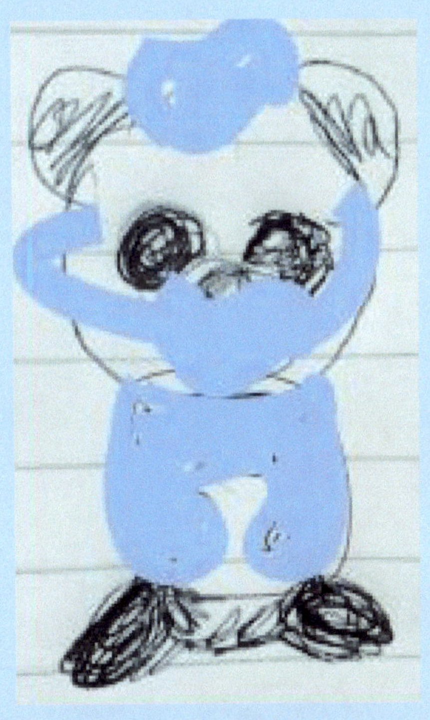

Ok Tuto.

Your checkup
is over.

Everything
looks great!

Don't forget to wear your
sunscreen so you don't
have any **flares**!

Do you know what a **flare**
is Tuto?

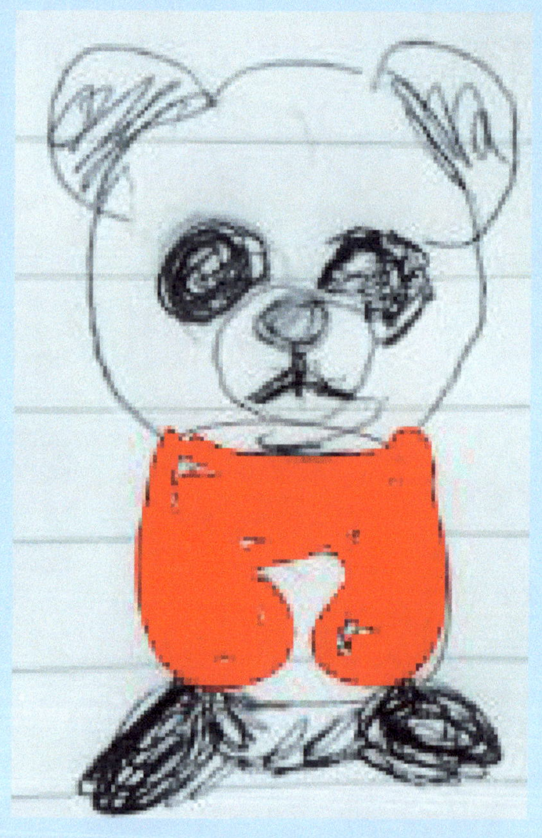

Yes, Doctor!

The End

Suggested Next steps

1. Continue learning.

If you find something about our story or any other diagnosis that interest you, don't ignore it. Research on your own and go on a quest for truth!

2. Continue sharing.

Much like love, knowledge is best when shared. Let others in on all you learn!

3. Continue hoping.

Rather you're having a hard time, had a hard time or heading for a hard time. Don't forget to keep hope!

www.ingramcontent.com/pod-product-compliance
Lightning Source LLC
Chambersburg PA
CBHW041804260726
48664CB00034B/297